Vegetarian Diet I

Amazing Super-Easy Recipe
Vegetarian Meals and Bo

America Best Recipes

Table of Contents

Breakfast

Chocolate Muffins

Prep time: 10 min Cooking Time: 12 min Serve: 2

Ingredients

¼ cup coconut oil

1/8 cup honey

1 egg

½ cup almond flour

1/8 cup cocoa powder

¼ teaspoon baking soda

1/8 teaspoon baking powder

1/6 cup almond milk

1/6 cup chocolate chips

Baking spray

1 1/2 cups of water

Instructions

Add melted coconut oil and honey to a large bowl and whisk to combine, until shiny and smooth.

6

Add the egg and whisk.

Add ½ cup almond flour, baking soda, baking powder, and cocoa powder. Whisk to combine.

Add the remaining almond milk and whisk to combine.

Stir in chocolate chips.

Spray a pressure cooker egg mold with baking spray and fill in the molds 3/4 with the muffin batter.

Add 1 1/2 cups of water to the Instant Pot and place the trivet inside.

Place the uncovered mold on top of the trivet.

Lock lid and seal the valve.

Cook on High Pressure for 12 minutes followed by a 10-minute natural pressure release.

Carefully open the lid, remove the mold.

Let it cool a bit and remove the muffins.

Sprinkle with powdered sugar and top with strawberry jam before serving if desired.

Nutrition Facts

Calories 404, Total Fat 27.5g, Saturated Fat 10.7g, Cholesterol 85mg, Sodium 206mg, Total Carbohydrate 36.2g, Dietary Fiber 5.6g, , Total Sugars 26.5g , Protein 11.3g

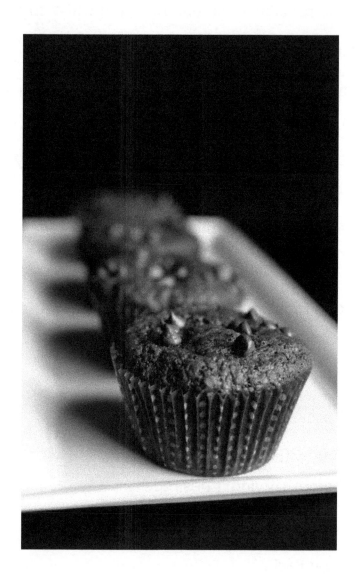

Pumpkin Chocolate Chip Quinoa Muffins
Prep time: 10 min Cooking Time: 10 min Serve: 2

Ingredients

1 egg

¼ cup canned pumpkin puree

2 tablespoons honey

¼ tablespoon coconut oil, melted

¼ teaspoon vanilla extract

¼ cup cooked quinoa

1/8 cup coconut flour

1 tablespoon baking powder

2 teaspoons pumpkin pie spice

1/4 teaspoon salt

1/3 cup mini chocolate chips

1 cup of water

Cooking spray

Instructions

In a large bowl whisk egg, pumpkin puree, honey, coconut oil, and vanilla extract until smooth.

Add quinoa, coconut flour, baking powder, salt, spice, and chocolate chips, then stir until combined.

Generously spray the 2 silicone molds with non-stick cooking spray. Using an ice cream scoop (about 1/4 cup), divide the batter into the molds.

Stack one of the filled molds on top of a trivet. Pour 1 cup of water into the Pressure Cooker Pot and place the trivet and filled silicone molds inside.

Lock lid in place and turn the valve to Sealing. Press the Pressure Cooker button and set the cook time for 10 minutes at High Pressure. When cooking is complete, use a Natural-release for 10 minutes and then release any remaining pressure.

Let the muffins cool if needed for handling.

Enjoy warm.

Store extras in the refrigerator. Delicious chilled or warmed up.

Nutrition Facts

Calories 234, Total Fat 6.4g, Saturated Fat 3g, Cholesterol 82mg , Sodium 349mg, Total Carbohydrate 41.2g, Dietary Fiber 3.2g Total Sugars 19.9g, Protein 6.6g

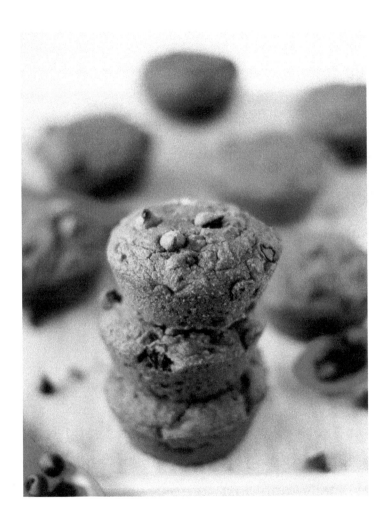

Baked Eggs with Creamy Collard Greens

Prep time: 05 min Cooking Time: 25 min Serve: 2

Ingredients

2 tablespoons avocado oil

½ tablespoon chopped onion

½ cup cottage cheese crumbled

½ cup collard greens

1 tablespoon coconut cream

Salt

Freshly ground black pepper

2 eggs

Chopped fresh basil

Instructions

Select Sauté on the Instant Pot and heat 1 tablespoon of the avocado oil. Add the onion and cook, stirring occasionally, until just softned, about 1 minute. Add the cottage cheese and cook, stirring occasionally, for 2 minutes. Add the remaining avocado oil and the collard greens and cook until the greens is wilted, about 5 minutes. Add the coconut cream and 1/2 teaspoon salt and cook until most of the liquid has been reduced, about 15 minutes. Add 1/4 teaspoon pepper and taste, adjusting seasoning as desired.

Press the Cancel button to reset the program. Make two wells in the collard greens and carefully crack 1 egg into each well. Lock lid in place and turn the valve to Sealing. Press the Pressure Cooker button and set the cook time for 1 minute at Low Pressure.

Turn the valve to Venting to release the steam quickly. When the steam stops, carefully remove the lid. Transfer each egg on a bed of collard greens to a plate, top with basil, if using, and more pepper, and serve .

Nutrition Facts

Calories144, Total Fat 8.6g, Saturated Fat 3.7g, Cholesterol 166mg Sodium 372mg, Total Carbohydrate 4g , Dietary Fiber 1.3g , Total Sugars 2.3g, Protein 13.3g

Ananas Quinoa

Prep time: 05 min Cooking Time: 05 min Serve: 2

Ingredients

½ tablespoon melted butter

1 cup soy milk

½ cup pineapple juice

½ cup quinoa

½ cup fresh pineapple diced

Raspberries

Instructions

Pour butter, soy milk, pineapple juice and quinoa into Instant Pot in that order. Swirl to make sure all quinoa are submerged.

Lock lid, making sure the vent is closed.

Using the display panel select the Manual function. Use the + /- keys and program the Instant Pot for 5 minutes.

When the time is up, let the pressure release naturally until the pin drops for about 15 minutes.

Stir in pineapple.

Serve with raspberries.

Nutrition Facts

Calories300, Total Fat 7.7g, Saturated Fat 2.4g, Cholesterol 8mg Sodium 89mg, Total Carbohydrate 47.6g, Dietary Fiber 4.7g , Total Sugars 14.1g, Protein 10.6g

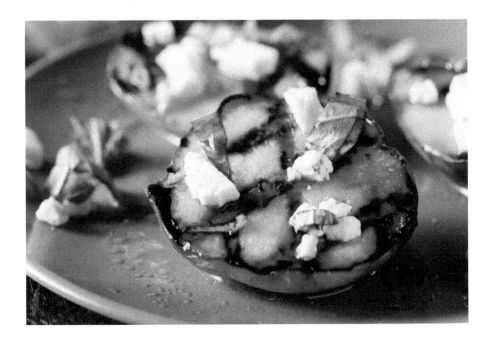

Blueberries Coconut Milk Yogurt

Prep time: 05 min Cooking Time: 14hr. Serve: 2

Ingredients

2 cups plain, sweetened coconut milk

1 1/2 tablespoon plain, dairy-free yogurt (soy, cashew, or almond)

1 teaspoon vanilla extract

1 pint fresh blueberries

1 tablespoon cashew roughly chopped

2 tablespoons maple syrup

Instructions

Add the coconut milk and yogurt to the inner pot. Stir well.

Lock lid in place and turn the valve to Sealing. Select Yogurt and set the cook time for 14 hours. When the cook time is complete, remove the lid and stir in the vanilla extract.

Allow the yogurt to cool slightly, and then transfer to a large, seal-able glass jar, and seal tightly. Place in the refrigerator to chill and thicken for a minimum of 4 hours.

To serve, transfer the chilled yogurt to serving bowls. Top each serving with 1/2 cup blueberries and chopped cashews, and then drizzle maple syrup over top

Nutrition Facts

Calories758, Total Fat 60.3g, Saturated Fat 51.2g, Cholesterol 0mg , Sodium 44mg, Total Carbohydrate 57.9g, Dietary Fiber 10.3g , Total Sugars 40.4g, Protein 8.2g

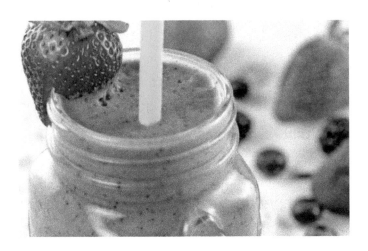

Sweet Potato Seasoning

½ teaspoon red chilli

Salt and pepper to taste

Instructions

Add 1½ cups water to into Instant Pot, add a vegetable steamer and spread out the Sweet potatoes.

Add all the tofu ingredients to a short Pyrex pan and toss to coat. Cover with foil and place on the sweet potatoes.

Mix the Spinach, water and garlic in a mixing bowl, transfer to a short Pyrex pan, cover with foil and place on top of the dish containing the tofu. Cook on High Pressure for 10 minutes. Let the pressure release naturally.

Once the pressure indicator goes down, remove the lid and carefully lift out the pan.

Toss the Sweet potatoes in a bowl with the red chilli, then add salt and pepper to taste. Serve in a bowl in layers or on a plate.

Nutrition Facts

Calories 176, Total Fat 2.9g, Saturated Fat 0.6g,Cholesterol 0mg, , Sodium 221mg, Total Carbohydrate 32.7g, Dietary Fiber 4.5g , Total Sugars 9.8g, Protein 7.6g

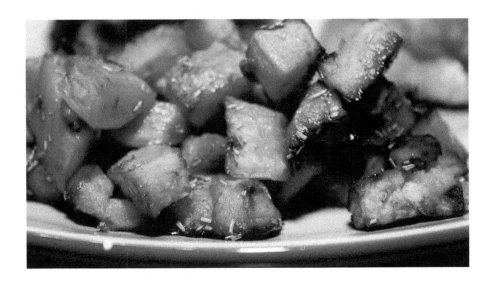

Herb & Cheese Omelet

Preparation Time: 6 minutes Cooking Time: 5 minutes
Servings: 2

Ingredients:

4 eggs

Salt and pepper to taste

2 tbsp. low-fat milk

1 tsp. chives, chopped

1 tbsp. parsley, chopped

½ cup goat cheese, crumbled

1 tsp. olive oil

Directions:

Beat the eggs in a bowl. Stir in the salt, pepper and milk. In a bowl, combine the chives, parsley and goat cheese. Cook the eggs for 3 minutes. Add the cheese mixture on top. Fold and serve.

Green Breakfast Salad

Preparation Time: 11 minutes Cooking time: 10 minutes

Servings: 4

Ingredients:

1 tablespoon lemon juice 4 red bell peppers 1 lettuce head, cut into strips Salt and black pepper to the taste 3 tablespoons coconut cream 2 tablespoons olive oil 1 ounces rocket leaves

Directions:

Place bell pepper in your air fryer's basket, cook at 400 degrees F for 10 minutes, transfer to a bowl, leave them aside to cool down, peel, cut them in strips and put them in a bowl. Add rocket leaves and lettuce strips and toss. In a bowl, mix oil with lemon juice, coconut cream, salt and pepper, whisk well, add over the salad, toss to coat, divide between plates and serve for breakfast. Enjoy!

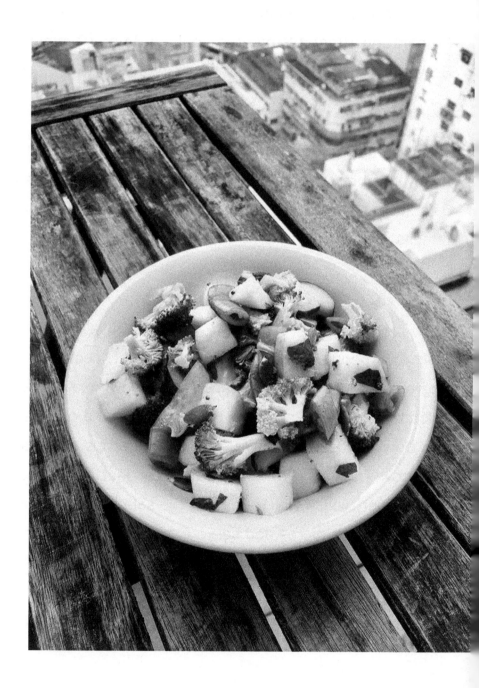

Wheat Quick Bread

Servings: 1 loaf Preparation Time: 10 mins Cooking Time: 20 mins

Ingredients:

1cup oats 1cup flour

1 cup soy milk

2 tsp. baking powder

1½ tbsp. agave syrup

1 tbsp. vegetable oil 1 tsp. Salt

Directions:

Preheat the oven to 450 degrees Fahrenheit. Blend the oatmeal to make oatmeal flour. Combine oatmeal flour, whole wheat flour, baking powder and salt. Spread the syrup in a separate bowl with vegetable oil, and then stir in the soy milk. Combine both the dry and wet mixtures and stir until they form a soft dough. Form the dough into a smooth round ball and place on a lightly oiled baking sheet. Bake in for 20 minutes, or until the bottom crust of loaf sounds hollow when tapped.

Sweet Pomegranate Porridge

Preparation time: 5 minutes Cooking time: 30 minutes Servings: 4

Ingredients:

2 Cups Oats 1 ½ Cups Water 1 ½ Cups Pomegranate Juice 2 Tablespoons Pomegranate Molasses

Directions:

Pour all ingredients into the instant pot and mix well. Seal the lid, and cook on high pressure for four minutes. Use a quick release, and serve warm.

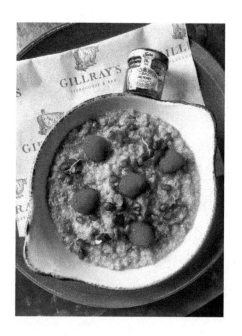

Lunch

Simple Roasted Broccoli and Cauliflower

Ingredients

cooking spray

1 tablespoon extra virgin olive oil

3 cloves garlic, minced

1/2 teaspoon sea salt

1/4 teaspoon ground black pepper

3 1/2 cups broccoli florets

2 1/2 cups cauliflower florets

1 tablespoon chopped fresh thyme

Directions:

Preheat your oven to 450 degrees F. Line a baking sheet with foil and grease with olive oil. Mix the olive oil, garlic, salt, and pepper in a bowl. Add in the cauliflower and tomatoes. Combine until well coated. Spread them out in a single layer on the baking sheet.

Roast in the oven until vegetables become caramelized for about 25 minutes. Top with the thyme. Simple

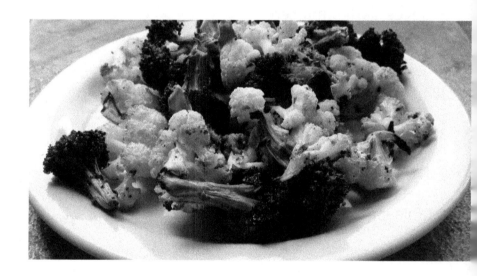

Simple Roasted Kale Artichoke Heart and Choy Sum Extra

Ingredients

1 tablespoon extra virgin olive oil

1/2 teaspoon sea salt

1/4 teaspoon ground black pepper

Main Ingredients

1 bunch of kale, rinsed and drained

1 cup canned artichoke hearts

1/2 medium Chinese flowery cabbage (choy sum), coarsely chopped

Directions:

Preheat your oven to 450 degrees F. Line a baking sheet with foil and grease with olive oil. Mix the extra ingredients thoroughly. Add in the main ingredients. Combine until well coated. Spread them out in a single layer on the baking sheet. Roast in the oven until vegetables become caramelized for about 25 minutes.

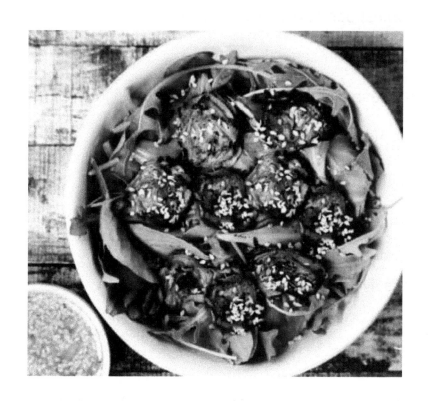

Roasted Spinach and Mustard Greens Extra

Ingredients

cooking spray

1 tablespoon extra virgin olive oil

1/2 teaspoon sea salt

1/4 teaspoon ground black pepper

Main Ingredients

5 baby carrots

1 bunch of spinach, rinsed and drained

1 bunch of mustard greens, rinsed and drained

Directions:

Preheat your oven to 450 degrees F. Line a baking sheet with foil and grease with olive oil. Mix the extra ingredients thoroughly. Add in the main ingredients. Combine until well coated. Spread them out in a single layer on the baking sheet. Roast in the oven until vegetables become caramelized for about 25 minutes.

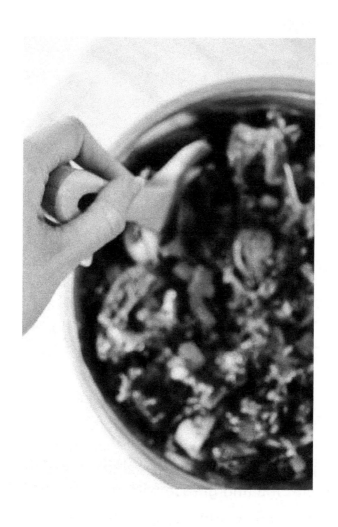

Roasted Kale and Bok Choy Extra

Ingredients

cooking spray

1 tablespoon extra virgin olive oil

1/2 teaspoon sea salt

1/4 teaspoon ground black pepper

Main Ingredients

1 bunch of kale, rinsed and drained

1 bunch of bok choy, rinsed, drained, and coarsely chopped

Directions:

Preheat your oven to 450 degrees F. Line a baking sheet with foil and grease with olive oil. Mix the extra ingredients thoroughly. Add in the main ingredients. Combine until well coated. Spread them out in a single layer on the baking sheet. Roast in the oven until vegetables become caramelized for about 25 minutes.

Roasted Lima Beans and Summer Squash

Ingredients

2 (15 ounces) cans lima beans, rinsed and drained

1/2 summer squash - peeled, seeded, and cut into 1-inch pieces

1 red onion, diced

1 sweet potato, peeled and cut into 1-inch cubes

2 large carrots, cut into 1 inch pieces

3 medium potatoes, cut into 1-inch pieces

3 tablespoons sesame oil Seasoning ingredients

1 teaspoon salt

1/2 teaspoon ground black pepper

1 teaspoon onion powder

2 teaspoon garlic powder

1 teaspoon ground fennel seeds

1 teaspoon dried rubbed sage

Garnishing Ingredients

2 green onions, chopped (optional)

Directions:

Preheat your oven to 350 degrees F. Grease your baking pan. Combine the beans, summer squash, onion, sweet potato, carrots, and russet potatoes on the prepared sheet pan. Drizzle with the oil and toss to coat. Combine the seasoning ingredients in a bowl. Sprinkle them over the vegetables on the pan and toss to coat with seasonings. Bake in the oven for 25 minutes. Stir frequently until vegetables are soft and lightly browned and beans are crisp, for about 20 to 25 minutes more. Season with more salt and black pepper to taste, top with the green onion before serving.

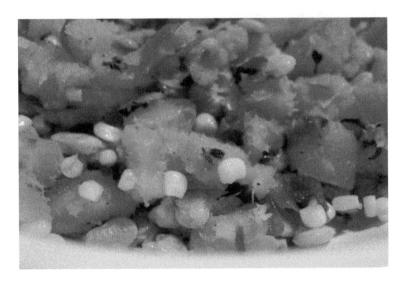

Spicy and Smoky Baked Brussels Sprouts and Red Beets

Ingredients

1 ½ cups Brussels sprouts, trimmed

1 cup large potato chunks

1 cup large red beets cut into chunks

1 ½ cup cauliflower florets

1 cup cubed red beets

1/2 cup red onion chunks

1 tsp. cumin

1 tsp. cayenne pepper

2 tablespoons extra-virgin olive oil

Salt and ground black pepper to taste

Directions:

Preheat your oven to 425 degrees F (220 degrees C). Set the rack to the second-lowest level in the oven. Pour some lightly salted water into a bowl. Submerge the Brussels sprouts in salted water for 15 minutes and drain. Place the rest of the ingredients together in a bowl. Spread the vegetables in a single layer onto a baking pan. Roast in the oven until the vegetables start to brown and cook through for about 45 minutes.

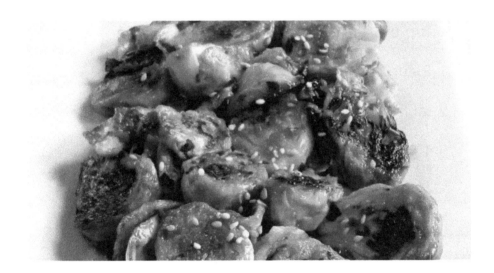

Baked Enoki and Mini Cabbage

Ingredients

1 ½ cups mini cabbage, trimmed

1 cup broccoli florets

1 cup enoki mushrooms, sliced

1 ½ cup cauliflower florets

1 cup oyster mushrooms

1/2 cup red onion chunks

2 tablespoons olive oil

Salt and ground black pepper to taste

Directions:

Preheat your oven to 425 degrees F (220 degrees C). Set the rack to the second-lowest level in the oven. Pour some lightly salted water into a bowl. Submerge the Brussels sprouts in salted water for 15 minutes and drain. Place the rest of the ingredients together in a bowl. Spread the vegetables in a single layer onto a

baking pan. Roast in the oven until the vegetables start to brown and cook through for about 45 minutes.

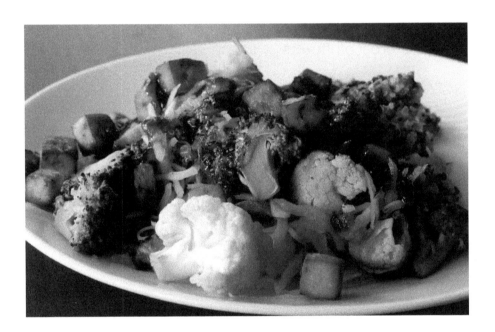

Roasted Spinach Brussels Sprouts and Broccoli

Ingredients

1   ½ cups Brussels sprouts, trimmed

1 cup spinach, coarsely chopped

1 cup romaine lettuce, coarsely chopped

1 ½ cup cauliflower florets

1 cup broccoli florets

1/2 cup red onion chunks

2 tablespoons extra-virgin olive oil

Sea salt and ground rainbow peppercorns to taste

¼ cup grated parmesan

Directions:

Preheat your oven to 425 degrees F (220 degrees C).
Set the rack to the second-lowest level in the oven.
Pour some lightly salted water into a bowl. Submerge
the Brussels sprouts in salted water for 15 minutes and
drain. Place the rest of the ingredients together in a
bowl. Spread the vegetables in a single layer onto a

baking pan. Roast in the oven until the vegetables start to brown and cook through for about 45 minutes.

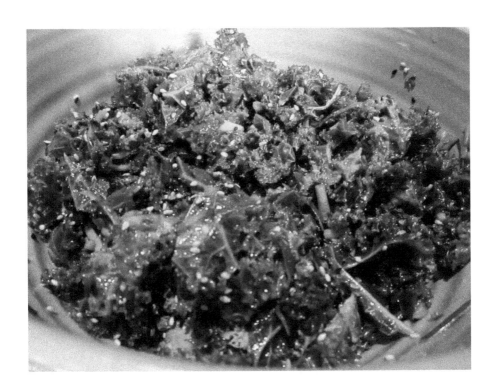

Roasted Mini Cabbage Rainbow Carrots & Bean Sprouts

Ingredients

1 ½ cups mini cabbage, trimmed

1 cup bean sprouts

1 cup large rainbow carrot chunks

1 ½ cup cauliflower florets

1 cup broccoli florets

1/2 cup red onion chunks

2 tablespoons canola oil

2 tbsp. Thai chili garlic paste

1 Thai basil salt and ground black pepper to taste

Directions:

Preheat your oven to 425 degrees F (220 degrees C). Set the rack to the second-lowest level in the oven. Pour some lightly salted water into a bowl. Submerge the mini cabbage in salted water for 15 minutes and drain. Place the rest of the ingredients together in a bowl. Spread the vegetables in a single layer onto a baking pan. Roast in the oven until the vegetables start to brown and cook through for about 45 minutes.

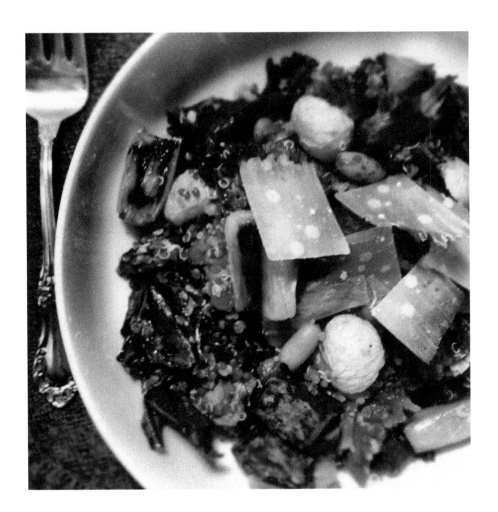

Roasted Mini Cabbage and Sweet Potato

Ingredients

1 ½ cups mini cabbage, trimmed

1 cup large potato chunks

1 cup large rainbow carrot chunks

1 ½ cup potato chunks

1 cup parsnips

1/2 cup red onion chunks

2 tablespoons extra-virgin olive oil

Sea salt Rainbow peppercorns to taste

1/4 cup cottage cheese

Directions:

Preheat your oven to 425 degrees F (220 degrees C). Set the rack to the second-lowest level in the oven. Pour some lightly salted water into a bowl. Submerge the mini cabbage in salted water for 15 minutes and drain. Place the rest of the ingredients together in a bowl. Spread the vegetables in a single layer onto a

baking pan. Roast in the oven until the vegetables start to brown and cook through for about 45 minutes.

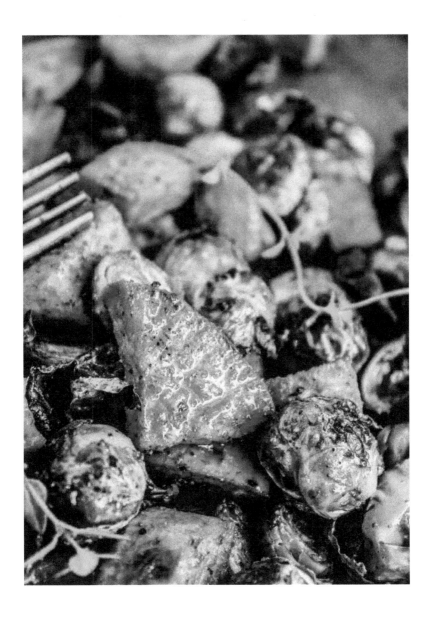

Soups and Salads

Bok Choy Soup
(Prep time: 05 min| Cooking Time: 10 min| Serve: 2)

Ingredients

2 cups of bok choy, diced

1 celery

1 bell pepper

1 potato, peeled and diced

1.5 cups of vegetable stock

½ cup of soy milk

Salt and pepper to taste

Instructions

Add diced bok choy, celery, potato, vegetable stock, and soy milk and bell pepper into Instant Pot.

Add salt and pepper to the mixture.

Turn the Instant Pot to the —Soup‖ function and let it cook. Alternatively, put everything in a pot and bring to boil and simmer until the celeriac and potato are soft.

When cool, puree it with an immersion blender like this one or put it in a High-speed blender.

Enjoy!

Nutrition Facts

Calories 131, Total Fat 1.6g, Saturated Fat 0.2g, Cholesterol 0mg, Sodium 131mg, Total Carbohydrate 26g, Dietary Fiber 3.6g, Total Sugars 7.5g, Protein 5.8g

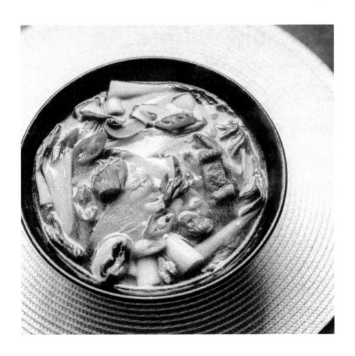

Spicy Peanut Soup with Potato and Spinach
(Prep time: 05 min| Cooking Time: 10 min| Serve: 2)

Ingredients

½ tablespoons butter

½ onion, diced

1 bell pepper, minced

1 teaspoon garlic, minced

1 potato, peeled and cubed

1 tomato

½ cup coconut milk

2 cups vegetable broth

1 teaspoon salt

½ teaspoon turmeric

1/8 cup chopped peanuts

1 teaspoon peanut butter

1 cup spinach, chopped

Instructions

Select the Sauté function to heat the instant Pot inner pot. When the pot displays —Hot‖, add butter, onion, and garlic. Sauté until the onion softens. Add the bell pepper, potato, tomatoes, coconut milk, broth, turmeric, peanuts, salt, and pepper. Stir them well. Lock lid in place and turn the valve to Sealing. Press the Pressure Cooker button and set the time to10 minutes. Once cooking is complete, turn the valve to the Venting position to release the pressure. When all the pressure is released, carefully remove the lid. Add spinach and peanut butter into the mixer. Use a standing blender or an immersion blender to puree the soup to a smooth, creamy consistency.

Serve.

Nutrition Facts

Calories 386, Total Fat 24.9g, Saturated Fat 15.9g, Cholesterol 8mg, Sodium 1992mg, Total Carbohydrate 32.6g, Dietary Fiber 7.1g, Total Sugars 9.6g, Protein 12.8g

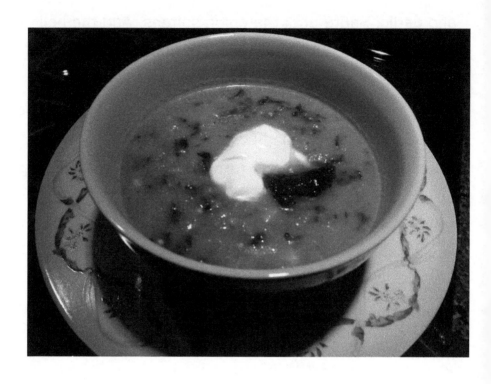

Parsnip Ginger Soup with Tofu and Kale
(Prep time: 10 min| Cooking Time: 20 min| Serve: 2)

Ingredients

½ tablespoon butter

1 small onion, diced

1 teaspoon ginger powder

1 teaspoon garlic powder

½ pound parsnip, cut into small coins

½ teaspoon cumin

½ teaspoon ground coriander

¼ teaspoon ground turmeric

1 1/2 cups of vegetable broth

½ cup of soy milk

½ teaspoon honey

½ fresh lime

1 cup tofu, diced into cubes

1 handful of fresh kale

Instructions

Set the Instant Pot to Sauté and add butter, add tofu cook it for 5 min. Keep aside.

After add onions. Cook for 5-10 minutes until the onion begins to soften.

Add the garlic and ginger powder to the pot and stir until fragrant.

Combine the parsnip, cumin, coriander powder, and turmeric powder in the Instant Pot. Stir well.

Pour in the broth and lock the lid. Turn the vent to seal, press Cancel, and manually cook on High Pressure for 5 minutes.

After 5 minutes, do a manual release.

Add the soy milk and honey if using to the Instant Pot. Allow the mixture to cool slightly, and then use an immersion blender or other mixer to puree until smooth. Season with salt, pepper, and a squeeze of lime.

Stir the fresh kale into the still, slightly warm soup. The kale should wilt on its own, but you can also warm it up together for the right temperature. Add the tofu, and enjoy!

Nutrition Facts

Calories 303, Total Fat 10.5g, Saturated Fat 3.3g, Cholesterol 8mg, Sodium

478mg, Total Carbohydrate 38.9g, Dietary Fiber 9.2g, Total Sugars 12.6g, Protein 18.1g

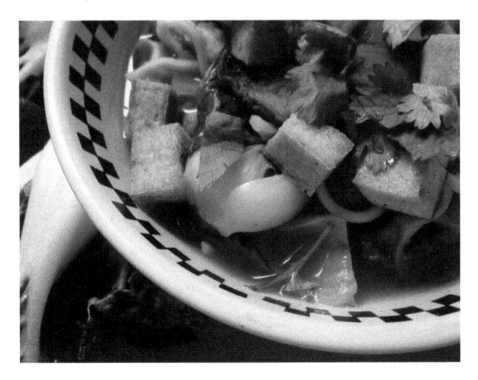

Mushroom Soup

(Prep time: 10 min| Cooking Time: 25 min| Serve: 2)

Ingredients

1 teaspoon avocado oil

½ medium onion, chopped

½ large leek stalk, chopped

½ large zucchini peeled & chopped

1 teaspoon garlic powder

8 ounces mushrooms sliced

½ teaspoon dried rosemary

¼ teaspoon ground pepper

1 1/2 cups vegetable broth

¼ teaspoon salt

½ cup almond milk

Instructions

Set the Instant Pot to Sauté mode. Heat the avocado oil, then add the onion, leek, and zucchini. Sauté the vegetables, occasionally stirring, until starting to soften, 3 to 4 minutes.

Add the garlic powder, mushrooms, rosemary, and pepper. Cook until the mushrooms are starting to release their liquid, 2 to 3 minutes. Stir in the broth and salt. Put the lid on the Instant Pot, close the steam vent, and set it to High Pressure using the Manual setting. Decrease the time to 10 minutes. It will take the Instant Pot about 10 minutes to reach pressure. Once the time is up, carefully release the steam using the Quick-release valve. Transfer half of the soup to the blender, add the almond milk, hold on the top and blend until almost smooth, stop the blender, and occasionally open the lid to release the steam. Transfer the pureed soup to a pot or bowl.

Nutrition Facts

Calories228, Total Fat 15.9g, Saturated Fat 13g, Cholesterol 0mg, Sodium 702mg, Total Carbohydrate 17.5g, Dietary Fiber 4.8g, Total Sugars 8.1g, Protein 9.3g

Seitan Stew with Barley
(Prep time: 10 min| Cooking Time: 20 min| Serve: 2)

Ingredients

1 teaspoon coconut oil

½ onion chopped

1 parsnip cut into thin half-circles

1 leek stalks diced

1 teaspoon garlic minced

1 teaspoon dried basil

½ teaspoons dried parsley

1 1/2 tablespoons tomato paste

2 cups vegetable broth

1 cup seitan

1 cup dry barley

½ teaspoon salt

½ teaspoon ground pepper

Instructions

Set the Instant Pot to Sauté mode. Heat the coconut oil, then add the onion, parsnips, and leek. Sauté the vegetables, occasionally stirring, until starting to soften, 3 to 4 minutes.

Add the garlic, basil, parsley, and tomato paste. Cook, constantly stirring, for 1 minute. Pour in the vegetable broth and stir to combine. Add the seitan, barley, and salt and pepper to the Instant Pot.

Put the lid on the Instant Pot, close the steam vent, and set it to High Pressure using the Manual setting. Set the time to 20 minutes. Once the time is expired, use Natural-release for 10 minutes, then quickly release.

Serve soup with salt and pepper to taste.

Nutrition Facts

Calories 376, Total Fat 5.8g, Saturated Fat 2.9g, Cholesterol 0mg, Sodium 1600mg, Total Carbohydrate 57.9g, Dietary Fiber 13.7g, Total Sugars 8.2g, Protein 23.5g

German Potato Salad

(Prep time: 15 min| Cooking Time: 15 min | serve: 2)

Ingredients

1 1/2 cups potatoes

1 small onion, diced

2 tablespoons water

3 tablespoons maple syrup

1 tablespoon olive oil

1/8 teaspoon salt

1/8 teaspoon ground black pepper

1 tablespoon chopped fresh basil

1 cup water

Instructions

Add 1 cup water to the Instant Pot. Place the trivet on the bottom of the pot and place the potatoes on the trivet. Lock the lid into place and make sure the nozzle is in the Sealing position. Use the Manual setting and set the timer for 12 minutes. Use the Quick Release method when the timer is up. Keep aside.

Pour oil, and select Sauté in Instant Pot. Add onion, and cook until browned. Add maple syrup, salt, and pepper to the Instant Pot. Add the potatoes and basil. Heat through, then transfer to a serving dish.

Enjoy.

Nutrition Facts

Calories 150, Total Fat 0.2g, Saturated Fat 0g, Cholesterol 0mg, Sodium 155mg, Total Carbohydrate 36.7g, Dietary Fiber 1.7g, Total Sugars 20.4g, Protein 1.6g

Creamy Avocado Egg Salad

(Prep time: 15 min| Cooking Time: 10 min | serve: 2)

Ingredients

2 eggs

½ large avocado, peeled and chopped

¼ cup seeded and chopped tomatoes

½ cup diced red onion

Salt and ground black pepper to taste

2 tablespoons mayonnaise

2 tablespoons coconut cream

1 tablespoon lemon juice

1 cup water

Instructions

Pour the water into the Instant Pot. Place a steamer basket or the trivet in the pot. Carefully arrange eggs in the steamer basket. Secure the lid on the Instant Pot.

Close the pressure-release valve. For hard-cooked eggs, select Manual and Cook at Low Pressure for 5 minutes. When cooking time is complete, use a Natural Release to depressurize. Remove the lid from the pot and gently place eggs in a bowl of cool water.

Chop eggs and transfer to a large bowl. Combine eggs, avocados, tomatoes, red onion, salt, and pepper in a bowl. Stir mayonnaise, coconut cream, lemon juice, and into egg mixture until evenly coated.

Nutrition Facts

Calories 286, Total Fat 22.8g, Saturated Fat 7.4g, Cholesterol 168mg, Sodium 175mg, Total Carbohydrate 12.7g, Dietary Fiber 4.6g, Total Sugars 4g, Protein 7.5g

Kale Pasta Salad

(Prep time: 15 min| Cooking Time: 10 min | serve: 2)

Ingredients

½ cup pasta

¼ cup kale, rinsed and torn into bite-size piece

½ cup crumbled goat cheese

1 small red onion, chopped

¼ cup Italian-style salad dressing

¼ teaspoon garlic powder

¼ lemon, juiced

½ teaspoon salt

½ teaspoon ground black pepper

1 cup water

Instructions

In Instant Pot. Add pasta and water. Cover the Instant Pot and lock it in. Set the Manual or Pressure Cook timer for 10 minutes. In a large bowl, combine the pasta, kale, cheese, red onion. Whisk together the salad dressing, garlic powder, lemon juice, salt, and pepper. Pour over salad and toss. Refrigerate for 2 hours and serve chilled.

Nutrition Facts

Calories 193, Total Fat 11.2g, Saturated Fat 3.1g, Cholesterol 27mg, Sodium 620mg, Total Carbohydrate 18.9g, Dietary Fiber 1.8g, Total Sugars 4.8g, Protein 4.9g

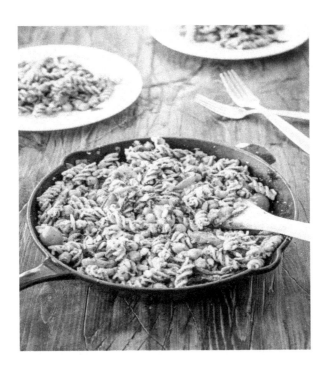

Garden Pasta Salad

(Prep time: 15 min| Cooking Time: 10 min | serve: 2)

Ingredients

½ cup uncooked spiral pasta

¼ cup thinly sliced carrots

1 stalk leek, chopped

½ cup chopped green bell pepper

¼ cup cucumber, peeled and thinly sliced

1 large tomato, diced

1/8 cup chopped onion

1 tablespoon Italian-style salad dressing

½ cup grated mozzarella cheese

1 cup water

Instructions

In Instant Pot. Add pasta and water. Cover the Instant Pot and lock it in.

Set the Manual or Pressure Cook timer for 10 minutes.

Mix chopped carrots, cucumber, green pepper, tomato, and onion in a large bowl. Combine cooled pasta and vegetables in a large bowl. Pour Italian dressing over mixture, add mozzarella cheese and mix well. Chill for 1 hour before serving.

Nutrition Facts

Calories 208, Total Fat 4.3g, Saturated Fat 1.2g, Cholesterol 4mg, Sodium 189mg, Total Carbohydrate 36.4g, Dietary Fiber 5.7g, Total Sugars 7.4g, Protein 6g

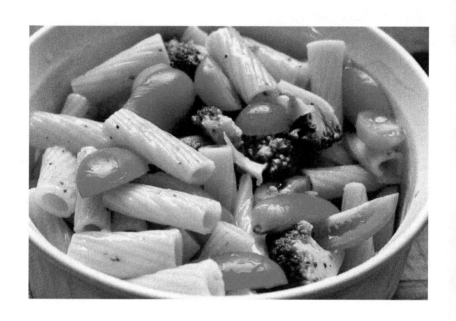

Dill Potato Salad

(Prep time: 15 min| Cooking Time: 15 min | serve: 2)

Ingredients

4 small red potatoes

2 tablespoons mayonnaise

¼ cup coconut cream

2 tablespoons dried dill

1 leek, chopped

Salt and ground black pepper to taste

1 cup water

Instructions

Add 1 cup water to the Instant Pot. Place the trivet on the bottom of the pot and place the potatoes on the trivet. Lock the lid into place and make sure the nozzle is in the Sealing position.

Use the Manual setting and set the timer for 12 minutes. Use the Quick Release method when the timer is up. Keep aside. 3. Combine mayonnaise, coconut cream, dill, and leek in a bowl and stir until blended. Season with salt and pepper to taste. Pour mayo mixture over potatoes and toss to coat evenly.

Adjust seasoning if necessary. Cover and refrigerate for at least 2 hours or overnight.

Nutrition Facts

Calories 326, Total Fat 12.6g, Saturated Fat 7.2g, Cholesterol 4mg, Sodium 137mg, Total Carbohydrate 47.1g, Dietary Fiber 5.5g, Total Sugars 5.8g, Protein 6.1g

Dinner

Turnips in Cilantro Gravy

(Prep time: 10 min |Cooking Time: 10 min | serve: 2)

Ingredients

7 turnips

¼ tablespoon cumin seeds

¼ tablespoon mustard seeds

1 tablespoon coconut oil

1/4 cup water

½ bunch fresh cilantro

Green chilies to taste

Salt to taste

½ teaspoon ginger powder

1 tablespoon tamarind pulp

Instructions

Grind cilantro, green chili, salt, ginger powder, and tamarind pulp using little or no water. Wash the turnips and make crisps cross slits till 3/4th length of turnips.

Stuff the ground cilantro paste into the turnips along the slits. Keep aside. Now press Sauté mode on High Pressure, add coconut oil.

Once the oil is hot, add cumin seeds and mustard seeds, fry well. Turn off Sauté mode. Add the stuffed turnips in one layer, then add the remaining cilantro paste. Add little water 1/4 cup to 1/2 cup. Mix gently (Optional). Make sure the vent is set to Sealing. Using the Manual function, set the cooker to Low Pressure for 5 minutes and quickly release after 2 minutes in Warm mode. Quickly release after 2 minutes in Warm mode. Serve with Rice.

Nutrition Facts

Calories 211, Total Fat 7.5g, Saturated Fat 5.9g, Cholesterol 0mg, Sodium 363mg, Total Carbohydrate

31.7g, Dietary Fiber 7.7g, Total Sugars 19.9g, Protein 4.3g

Bell Peppers & Sweet Potato Stir Fry

(Prep time: 5 min |Cooking Time: 15 min | serve: 2)

Ingredients

½ tablespoon avocado oil

1 bell pepper, cut into long pieces

2 sweet potatoes, cut into small pieces.

¼ teaspoon cumin seeds

1 teaspoon garlic powder

¼ tablespoon lemon juice

Basil to garnish

1/8 teaspoon turmeric powder

¼ teaspoon red chili powder

½ teaspoon coriander powder

½ teaspoon salt

Instructions

Put Instant Pot to Sauté mode and add avocado oil in it. Add cumin and garlic powder. Once the cumin and garlic powder turns golden brown, add the cut bell peppers, sweet potatoes, turmeric powder, coriander powder, red chili powder, and salt. Mix well. Sprinkle water with your hand. Change the Instant Pot setting to Manual mode or Pressure Cook mode at High Pressure for 2 minutes. Make sure the valve is Sealing. When the Instant Pot beeps, let the pressure release naturally. The veggies would be cooked. If they are watery, change the Instant Pot setting to Sauté mode and stir until you get the desired consistency. Stir in the lemon juice and mix well. Garnish with fresh basil and enjoy.

Nutrition Facts

Calories 209, Total Fat 1g, Saturated Fat 0.2g, Cholesterol 0mg, Sodium 601mg, Total Carbohydrate 48.1g, Dietary Fiber 7.5g, Total Sugars 4.2g, Protein 3.4g

Cauliflower Stir-Fry

(Prep time: 10 min |Cooking Time: 5 min | serve: 2)

Ingredients

½ tablespoon coconut oil

1 small onion, sliced thin

½ cup diagonally sliced zucchini

1 cup cauliflower florets

1 cup green peas

½ large red bell pepper, cut into strips

½ tablespoon reduced-sodium soy sauce

1 teaspoon minced garlic

1 teaspoon ginger, crushed

1 teaspoon sesame seed, toasted

Instructions

Put Instant Pot to Sauté mode and add coconut oil in it.
Add onion and minced garlic, and crushed ginger. Once

the onion turns golden brown, add the cut bell peppers, zucchini, cauliflower, green peas. Mix well. Sprinkle water and soy sauce with your hand. Change the Instant Pot setting to Manual mode or Pressure Cook mode at High Pressure for 2 minutes. Make sure the valve is in the —Sealing‖. Garnish with sesame seed and enjoy.

Nutrition Facts

Calories145, Total Fat 4.7g, Saturated Fat 3.1g, Cholesterol 0mg, Sodium 174mg, Total Carbohydrate

21.4g, Dietary Fiber 6.8g, Total Sugars 8.9g, Protein 6.6g

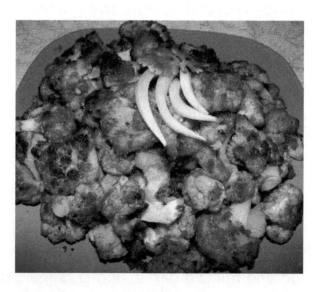

Easy Sweet Potato Asparagus

(Prep time: 5min |Cooking Time: 10 min | serve: 2)

Ingredients

½ tablespoon coconut oil

¼ teaspoon cumin seeds

½ teaspoon garlic powder

1 green chili, chopped

1 cup asparagus, chopped in 1/2-inch pieces

½ sweet potato, cubed into small pieces

1 teaspoon coriander powder

1/8 teaspoon turmeric powder

1/8 teaspoon red chili powder

½ teaspoon salt

½ teaspoon dry mango

Instructions

Start the Instant Pot on Sauté mode, heat it and then add coconut oil. Heating the pot first helps later. Then add cumin seeds, garlic powder, and green chili. When the cumin seeds start to splutter, add chopped asparagus and sweet potatoes. Add turmeric

powder, red chili powder, coriander powder, and salt and mix properly. Sprinkle water with your hand. Close the Instant Pot lid, and change the setting to Manual mode for 2 minutes. When the Instant Pot beeps, let the pressure release naturally. Mix in the dry mango powder. Served with roti.

Nutrition Facts

Calories 98, Total Fat 3.7g, Saturated Fat 3g, Cholesterol 0mg, Sodium 597mg, Total Carbohydrate 16.3g, Dietary Fiber 3.5g, Total Sugars 4.2g, Protein 2.3g

Ginger Veggie Stir-Fry

(Prep time: 5min |Cooking Time: 10 min | serve: 2)

Ingredients

½ tablespoon corn-starch

2 teaspoons garlic powder

2 teaspoons ginger powder

1/4 cup olive oil, divided

1 small head of broccoli, cut into florets

1/2 cup snow peas

3/4 cup julienned carrots

1/2 cup halved green beans

2 tablespoons soy sauce

2 1/2 tablespoons water

1/4 cup chopped onion

½ tablespoon salt

Instructions

In a large bowl, blend corn-starch, garlic, 1 teaspoon ginger, and 2 tablespoons olive oil until cornstarch is dissolved. Mix in broccoli, snow peas, carrots, and green beans, tossing to coat lightly. 2. Start the Instant Pot on Sauté mode, heat it, and then add coconut oil. Put all vegetables in the pot and sauté for 2 minutes, then add soy sauce and water. Mix well.

Close the Instant Pot lid, and change the setting to Manual mode for 5 minutes.

When the Instant Pot beeps, let the pressure release naturally. Serve.

Nutrition Facts

Calories 321, Total Fat 25.6g, Saturated Fat 3.7g, Cholesterol 0mg, Sodium 2693mg, Total Carbohydrate 18g, Dietary Fiber 4.3g, Total Sugars 6g, Protein 4.7g

Red Cabbage Coleslaw

Ingredients

¼ of a large red cabbage, shredded with a knife or mandolin

1 large carrot, peeled and julienned

½ medium white onion, thinly sliced

Dressing:

3 tablespoons aquafaba (chickpea cooking liquid)

½ cup canola oil

1 tablespoon apple cider vinegar

2 tablespoons lemon juice

2 tablespoons honey

½ teaspoon sea salt, or more to taste

Directions:

Combine the vegetables in a bowl. In a blender, add the aquafaba and slowly drizzle in the oil. Add the remaining dressing ingredients and blend. Pour this dressing over the vegetables and toss to combine. Taste and add salt.

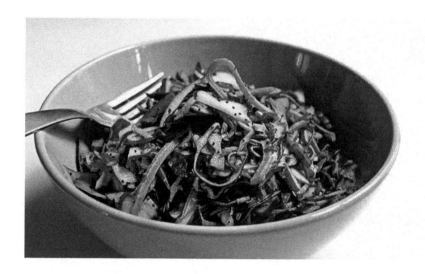

Vegetarian Macaroni and Cheese

Ingredients

3 1/2 cups elbow macaroni

1/2 cup butter

1/2 cup flour

3 1/2 cups boiling water

1-2 tsp. sea salt

2 Tbsp. soy sauce

1 1/2 tsp. garlic powder

Pinch of turmeric

1/4 cup olive oil

1 cup nutritional yeast flakes Spanish Paprika, to taste

Directions:

Preheat your oven to 350°F. Cook the elbow macaroni according to the package instructions. Drain the noodles. In a pan, heat the vegan margarine on low until melted. Add and whisk the flour. Continue whisking and increase to medium heat until smooth and bubbly. Add and whisk in the boiling water, salt, soy sauce, garlic powder, and turmeric. Continue to whisk until dissolved. Once thick and bubbly, whisk in the oil and the yeast flakes. Mix 3/4 of the sauce with the noodles and place in a baking dish. Pour the remaining sauce and season with the paprika. Bake for 15 minutes. Broil until crisp for a few min.

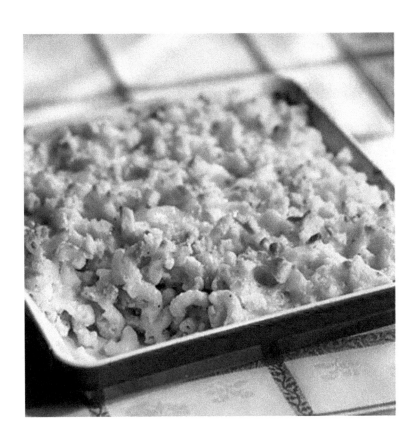

Vegetarian Pizza

Ingredients

1 piece vegan naan (Indian flatbread)

2 Tbsp. tomato sauce

1/4 cup shredded mozzarella

1/4 cup chopped fresh button mushrooms

3 thin tomato slices

2 vegan meatballs Quorn, thawed (if frozen) and cut into small pieces

1 tsp. vegan Parmesan

Pinch of dried basil

Pinch of dried oregano

½ tsp. sea salt

Directions:

Preheat your oven to 350ºF. Place the naan on a baking pan. Layer the sauce evenly over the top and sprinkle with half the vegan mozzarella shreds. Add in the mushrooms, tomato slices, and vegan meatball pieces. Layer with the rest of the vegan mozzarella shreds. Lightly season with the vegan Parmesan, basil, and oregano. Bake for 25 minutes.

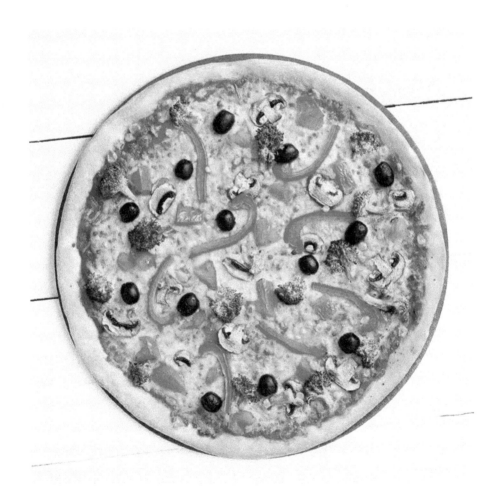

Tofu Stir Fry

Ingredients

1 package firm tofu, drained and mashed

Juice of 1/2 lemon

1/2 tsp. salt

1/2 tsp. turmeric

1 Tbsp. extra virgin olive oil

1/4 cup diced jalapeno

1/4 cup diced red onion

3 clove garlic, minced

1 Tbsp. chopped flat-leaf parsley

1 Tbsp. vegan bacon bits (optional)

Pepper, to taste (optional)

Directions:

In a bowl, mix the crumbled tofu, lemon juice, salt, and turmeric thoroughly. Heat the oil over medium heat and add the jalapeno, onion, and garlic. Stir fry for 2 1/2 minutes, or until just softened. Add the tofu mixture and cook for 15 minutes. Garnish with parsley, soy bacon pieces, and pepper.

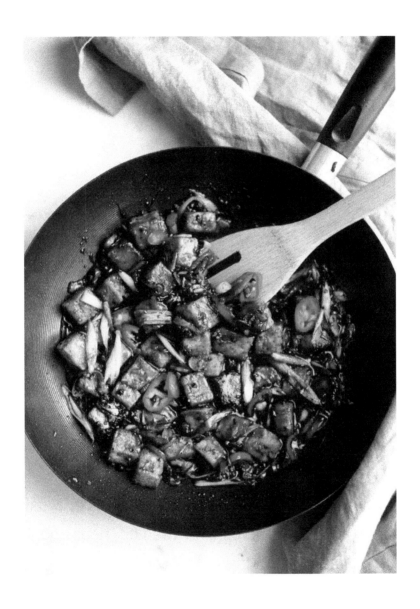

Simple Watercress Stir Fry

Ingredients

1 package firm watercress, rinsed and drained

Juice of 1/2 lemon

1/2 tsp. salt

1 Tbsp. extra virgin olive oil

1/4 cup diced green pepper

1/4 cup diced red onion

3 clove garlic, minced

1 Tbsp. chopped flat-leaf parsley

1 Tbsp. vegan bacon bits (optional)

Pepper, to taste (optional)

Directions:

In a bowl, mix the watercress, lemon juice, & salt thoroughly. Heat the oil over medium heat and add the pepper, onion, and garlic. Stir fry for 2 1/2 minutes, or until just softened. Add the tofu mixture and cook for

15 minutes. Garnish with parsley, soy bacon pieces, and pepper.

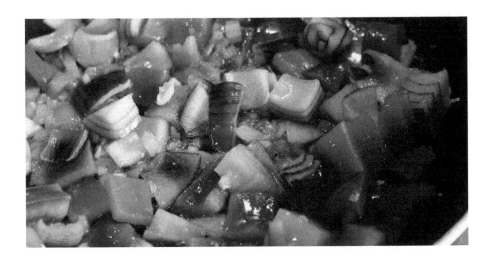

Sweets

Vegan Chocolate Peanut Butter Cookies

Vegan Chocolate Peanut Butter Cookies are healthy coconut flour vegan cookies with a shortbread crunchy and sandy texture made with only 4 ingredients.

Prep Time: 10 mins Cook Time: 12 mins Total Time: 22 mins

Ingredients

1 cup Natural Peanut butter fresh, runny 1/4 cup Coconut Flour sifted, no lumps

2 tablespoons unsweetened cocoa powder

1/4 cup sugar-free natural liquid sweetener or maple syrup

Instructions

Preheat oven to 180C (356F).

Prepare a cookie rack covered with parchment paper. Set aside. In a food processor with the S blade attachment, add all the ingredients, order doesn't matter. Process on medium speed for about 1 minute or until all the ingredients come together into a ball.

Stop the food processor, gather the ingredients together to form a ball and split in 8 even pieces.

Roll each piece into a cookie ball, place each ball on the prepared cookie rack leaving half thumb space between each cookies. The cookies won't spread so you don't have to leave too much space. If the dough is too dry or crumbly, you can oil your hands with a tiny amount of coconut oil to make the rolling easier.

Bake for 10-12 minutes.

Cool down on a cookie rack. I used a large spatula that I slide under the cookie to gently transfer the cookies one by one to the rack without breaking them.

When cool down, decorate with sugar free melted dark chocolate and chop peanuts. Place the cookies in the freezer for a few minutes to quickly set the melted chocolate if needed.

Store up to 3 weeks in a cookie jar.

Nutrition Info

Calories 218 Calories from Fat 140 Fat 15.6g24%

Saturated Fat 2.4g Carbohydrates 10.6g Fiber 5.2g22% Sugar 2.6g3% Protein 9.3g

Keto Gingerbread cookies vegan and gluten-free

Keto Gingerbread cookies an easy healthy gluten-free cookie recipe without molasses. A delicious crispy Christmas cookie for kids or cookie lovers.

Prep Time: 10 mins Cook Time: 20 mins Total Time: 50 mins

Ingredients

Dry ingredients

2 cup Almond Flour or almond meal 1/2 cup Erythritol or golden monk fruit 1 teaspoon Ground ginger

1/2 tablespoon Ground cinnamon

1 teaspoon Baking Powder or 1/2 teaspoon baking soda 1/4 teaspoon ground cloves

Wet ingredients

1 large Egg or 1 tablespoon chia seed + 3 tablespoons water 1/4 cup Coconut oil melted or butter

1 teaspoon Vanilla extract

1 tablespoon black strap molasse - optional, recipe work without it but great iron boost for vegan

Keto royal icing

1 cup sugar free icing sugar

1-2 tablespoon Unsweetened Almond Milk 1/4 teaspoon guar gum

Instructions

Preheat oven to 180°C (350°F) and line two cookie baking sheets with parchment paper. Set aside.

If you are vegan and don't want to use an egg, add chia seed and water in a small bowl. Stir. Set aside 10 minutes until it forms a gel.

In a large mixing bowl, combine the dry ingredients: almond flour, erythritol, and spices.

Add the beaten egg (or chia seed gel if keto vegan), melted coconut oil, molasses (optional!), and vanilla extract.

Combine with a spatula first, then use your hands and knead the dough until it comes together.

Divide the dough into two balls of the same size. Wrap each ball tightly into plastic wrap, roughly flatten into a thick disc and refrigerate both discs for 1 hour.

Remove the dough discs from the fridge, unwrap one disc and place it in the center of two parchment paper pieces.

Roll out the dough into a 1/2 inch thickness (for thicker cookies) or 1/4 inch thick (for thinner cookies).

Use a gingerbread man cookie cutter shape to cut out cookies - I made 6 cookies in each half-disc of dough, so 12 in total. My tip: use a small knife or spatula to lift the shaped cookie and transfer it onto the prepared baking cookie sheets.

Gather up the leftover dough into a ball and re-roll to form more cookies. You should be able to shape 12 large gingerbread cookies with the entire recipe, depending on your cookie cutter size.

Bake your cookies for 12-14 minutes max or until the border are golden brown.

Remove from the oven, cool down 5 minutes on the baking sheet, then gently transfer into a cooling rack. I recommend using a spatula that you slide under each cookie to transfer them gently. They will look soft, and that is ok! They will firm up with time. Cool them down for at least 20 minutes. Be patient; the cookies will get very crunchy with time! Trust me, after a few hours. You won't believe how crunchy and flavorsome they get! The gingerbread flavor will also enhance after 24 hours.

Store up to 2 weeks in a cookie jar, in the pantry.

Keto royal icing

Combine sugar-free icing powder with almond milk and guar gum until it forms a white paste.

Use a piping bag to pipe shapes on the cookies.

Dry at room temperature. It can take up to 48 hours for the decorations to harden.

Nutrition Info

Calories 138

Calories from Fat 100 Fat 11.1g Carbohydrates 5.1g Fiber 2.6g Protein 4.2g

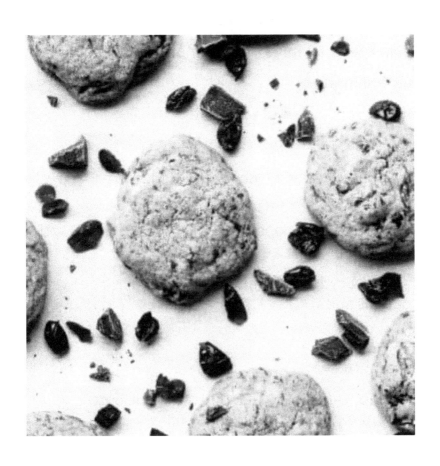

Keto no-bake cookies

Keto no-bake cookies are low carb peanut butter chocolate cookies packed with healthy coconut oil, flaxseed meal, and walnuts.

Prep Time: 10 mins Total Time: 30 mins

Ingredients

Dry ingredients

1 cup Almond Flour

1 cup unsweetened desiccated coconut 1 cup Walnuts , roughly chopped

2 1/2 tablespoons unsweetened cocoa powder 2 tablespoons Flaxseed meal

1/3 cup Erythritol or if paleo (not sugar free) you can use coconut sugar

Wet ingredients

3/4 cup Natural Peanut butter or nut butter you like 1/4 cup + 2 tablespoons Coconut oil

1 teaspoon Vanilla essence Chocolate glazing

1/2 cup Sugar-free Chocolate Chips or stevia sweetened chocolate

1/3 cup Coconut cream - thick part from top of can

2-4 drops stevia liquid optional, adjust regarding desired sweetness

Instructions

Line parchment paper on one or two plates. Make sure the plates fit in your freezer as you must freeze these cookies to set.

You may need more plates depending on your plate size. Set aside.

In a large mixing bowl, add all the dry ingredients EXCEPT the sugar-free sweetener (erythritol).

Stir to combine. Set aside.

In another mixing bowl, add peanut butter, coconut oil, vanilla, and erythritol. Microwave by 30 seconds bursts, stirring in between. Repeat until the coconut oil is fully melted and all the ingredients are combined. It should not take more than 1 minute 30 seconds.

If you don't have a microwave available, bring the ingredients into a small saucepan, warm under medium heat, stirring all the time until it forms a consistent mixture.

Stir in the peanut butter mixture onto the dry ingredients. Make sure the liquid covers all the dry ingredients, the batter will be quite wet and that's what you want.

Scoop out some cookie dough onto the prepared plate covered with parchment paper. You should be able to divide the batter into 12 large cookies.

Spread the dough with the back of a spoon to form a cookie shape.

Freeze for 20 minutes, until the cookies are hard. Meanwhile, prepare the chocolate glazing.

Chocolate glazing

In a mixing bowl add the sugar-free chocolate chips, coconut cream, and stevia drops. Microwave by 30 seconds bursts as you did before until the chocolate is fully melted. It will create a slightly thick chocolate cream.

Remove the cookies from the freezer.

Scoop out some of the chocolate glazing in the middle of each cookie and spread with the back of the spoon. Repeat for each cookie, until no more glazing left.

Decorate each no-bake keto cookie by adding walnuts halves in the center.

Return to the freezer 2-3 minutes to set the glazing. Enjoy your no-bake cookies!

This recipe makes about 12 large no-bake cookies.

Storage: They must be stored in an airtight container in the fridge or they will soften even melt during summer. Store up to 3-4 weeks in the fridge. You can also freeze these cookies and defrost 1 hour before eating.

Nutrition Info

Calories 194 Calories from Fat 152 Fat 16.9g26%

Carbohydrates 8.2g Fiber 3.3g14% Sugar 3.6g4% Protein 4.9g

Coconut flour cookies no sugar

Don't blow your diet this Christmas! Whatever you eat keto, low carb, paleo or vegan, these coconut flour cookies have no sugar. It's the healthy Christmas cookies you need to make everyone happy.

Prep Time: 15 mins Cook Time: 8 mins Total Time: 23 mins 12 cookies

Ingredients

Decoration

3/4 cup Coconut Flour

1/3 cup Coconut oil solid, not melted +/- 1 tablespoon (add if the dough is too crumbly)

1/4 cup Erythritol - monk fruit sugar or erythritol 1/4 teaspoon Vanilla extract

1 large Egg - at room temperature, or 1 tablespoon of peanut butter if vegan keto

1/3 cup Sugar-free Dark Chocolate I used stevia chocolate 1 tablespoon Pumpkin seeds crushed

1 teaspoon unsweetened desiccated coconut Optional - to sprinkle on top before baking

1 tablespoon Coconut Flour

Instructions

Preheat oven to fan-bake 180°C (350°F). Prepare a cookie tray, cover with parchment paper. Set aside.

Place all the ingredients in a bowl, beat with an electric beater until it forms a crumble. It should not take more than 20 seconds. If you don't have an electric beater you can also press/rub the dough with your hands until it forms a crumb - just a bit messier!

Assemble the crumb with your hands to form a cookie dough ball and transfer the ball onto a piece of plastic wrap. It's a crumbly dough, that's normal, press firmly with your hands to gather the pieces together and firmly wrap the batter to form a ball. If it really doesn't come together after you kneaded the dough for 1 minute, add slightly more coconut oil - up to 1 tablespoon max. Refrigerate for 15 minutes to firm up.

Remove from the fridge, open the plastic wrap, the dough will be firm but still crumbly when you take some in your hands that is ok. The more you knead the dough the easier it gets to form balls as the coconut oil softens.

Roll 1 tablespoon of dough into a ball, pressing the dough firmly in your hands. Place the balls onto the prepared baking sheet. If you want to make crescent-shaped cookies. First, shape the ball into a cylinder, slightly pinch the middle to form a crescent shape. The fastest will be to simply flatten the ball with a fork to form lovely round shortbread cookies. Repeat with remaining dough until you form 12 cookies.

If you like, sprinkle extra coconut flour on top of the cookies before baking.

Bake until light golden brown on the sides 6 to 8 minutes. The cookies will remain very soft at this stage and that is normal, don't touch them or don't try to remove them from the tray, they firm up when fully cool down.

Cool down on the baking sheet for about 30 minutes until it reaches room temperature. As it cools down, the coconut oil hardens and creates crispy crumbly shortbread cookies. I usually place my baking sheet outside in summer to cool down in fresh air quickly or near an open window.

Decorate with a drizzle of melted sugar-free chocolate if you like. I used dark chocolate sweetened with stevia.

Nutrition Info

Calories 208 Calories from Fat 175 Fat 19.4g Carbohydrates 6g Fiber 3.3g Sugar 2g2% Protein 2.5g

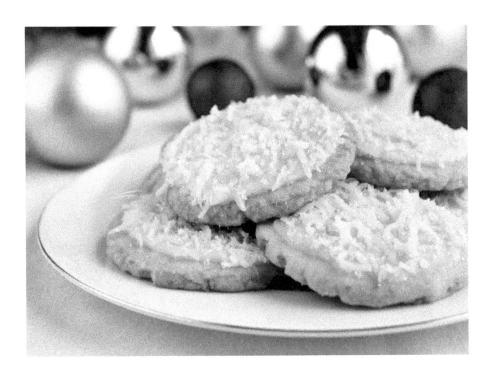

Low carb lemon cookies

Low carb lemon cookies are easy, healthy soft buttery cookies, with no butter and a bursting lemon juice flavor. 100 % Vegan + Keto + Gluten free these healthy lemon cookies with almond flour suit all diet.

Prep Time: 10 mins Cook Time: 15 mins Total Time: 55 mins

Ingredients

Dry ingredients

1 1/3 cup Almond Flour

2 tablespoons Coconut Flour

1/4 cup Erythritol - can go up to 1/3 cup for a sweeter flavor 1/2 teaspoon Baking soda

Liquid ingredients

1/4 cup Lemon Juice fresh or organic 1/4 cup Coconut oil

1 tablespoon Lemon Zest - optional Sugar-free lemon glazing

1/4 cup Sugar-free powdered sweetener 2 teaspoons Lemon Juice

1 teaspoon Coconut oil , melted

1 tablespoon Lemon Zest , optional, to decorate

Instructions

Preheat oven to 180°C (350°F). Line a cookie tray with parchment paper. Set aside.

In a medium mixing bowl, combine all the dry ingredients: almond flour, coconut flour, sugar-free crystal sweetener and baking soda. Set aside.

In a small mixing bowl, add coconut oil and lemon juice. Microwave for 30 seconds, stir and repeat until the coconut oil is fully melted. Otherwise, place the ingredients in a saucepan warm on medium heat. Remove from heat when the coconut oil is melted.

Pour liquid onto dry ingredients, add lemon zest if desired, and combine until it forms a cookie dough. You should be able to shape a ball. The batter should be soft, buttery, and not dry. If dry, adjust with 1-2 teaspoon of water but you shouldn't have to.

Refrigerate for 10 minutes, wrapped in a piece of plastic wrap or in the mixing bowl covered with silicone lid.

Remove the dough from the fridge and shape 8 even cookie dough balls. You can weigh the dough if you want precision.

Roll each ball in your hands to shape smooth cookie dough balls.

Place each ball on the cookie tray leaving a thumb-size space between each ball. The cookies won't expand in the oven so you don't have to leave a big space between them.

Press the balls slightly with your hand palm to flatten cookies. Don't flatten too much or the sides will form cracks and they won't be as soft and moist. The thicker, the moister!

Bake for 15 minutes or until golden on sides. The middle will stay slightly soft and that is the texture you want.

Remove the cookie tray from the oven and cool down on the tray for 20 minutes before transferring on the rack to cool down to room temperature. Don't touch the cookies during the first 20 minutes, they are soft and need time to firm up.

Prepare the sugar-free lemon glazing

In a small mixing bowl, combine the sugar-free powdered sweetener, coconut oil, and lemon juice. Play with the texture, adding more sweetener, 1 teaspoon at a time for a thicker glazing or more lemon juice for a thinner glazing.

Drizzle the glazing onto the cold cookies. Don't decorate warm or lukewarm cookies or the glazing will melt and be absorbed by the cookie dough.

For a lovely, white glazing, place the cookies 2 minutes in the

freezer just after adding the glazing. This step sets the glazing fast and makes beautiful cookie decorations.

Sprinkle lemon zest on top if desired.

Store the lemon cookies in an airtight container for up to 3 days in the pantry or in the fridge if you prefer your cookies firm.

Nutrition Info

Calories 194 Calories from Fat 102 Fat 11.3g17% Carbohydrates 6.6g2% Fiber 2.4g10% Protein 3.4g

Quick Cherry Crisp

Prep time: 25 min Cooking Time: 25 min serve: 2

Ingredients

¼ cup honey ½ tablespoon corn-starch

2 cups red cherries ½ cup crumbled shortbread cookies

1 tablespoon butter or margarine, melted

1/8 cup chopped almonds, toasted

Ice cream (optional)

Instructions

In a small bowl, combine honey and cornstarch. In an instant pot, sprinkle corn-starch mixture over cherries; stir to combine. Cover your Instant Pot, set the vent to Sealing, select the manual or pressure cook button, select high pressure and set the timer to 2 minutes.

When done allow the pot to undergo natural pressure release for 15 mins 10 minutes or until thickened and bubbly.

Meanwhile, in a medium bowl, thoroughly combine crumbled cookies, butter, and nuts

Divide cherry mixture among four dessert dishes. Sprinkle cookie mixture over cherry mixture. If desired, serve with ice cream.

Chocolate Chip Cheesecake

Prep time: 25 min Cooking Time: 25 min serve: 2

Ingredients

½ cup graham cracker crumbs

1 tablespoon honey

½ cup unsweetened cocoa powder

½ cup butter, melted

½ cup cream cheese

1 cup sweetened condensed milk

1 egg

1 teaspoon vanilla extract

½ cup mini semi-sweet chocolate chips

1 teaspoon coconut flour

Instructions

Mix graham cracker crumbs, honey, butter and cocoa. Press onto bottom and up the sides of a 9 inch spring form pan. Set crust aside.

Beat cream cheese until smooth. Gradually add sweetened condensed milk; beat well. Add vanilla and egg, and beat on medium speed until smooth. Toss 1/3 of the miniature chocolate chips with the 1 teaspoon coconut flour to coat (this keeps them from sinking to the bottom of the cake). Mix into cheese mixture. Pour into prepared crust. Sprinkle top with remaining chocolate chips.

Pour the water into the Instant Pot Insert, and place a trivet with the covered brownie cake tin into the Instant Pot.

Cover your Instant Pot, set the vent to Sealing, select the manual or pressure cook button, select high pressure and set the timer to 30 minutes.

When done allow the pot to undergo natural pressure release for 15 mins.

Refrigerate before removing sides of pan. Keep cake refrigerated until time to serve.

Nutrition Facts

Calories 418, Total Fat 43.3g, Saturated Fat 26.4g, Cholesterol 160mg, Sodium 458mg, Total Carbohydrate 61.5g, Dietary Fiber 4.3g, Total Sugars 48.4g, Protein 12.7g

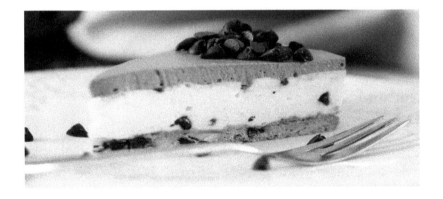

Peanut Butter Fudge

Prep time: 25 min Cooking Time: 25 min serve: 2

Ingredients

1 tablespoon honey

1/8 cup coconut milk

½ cup marshmallow crème

1 cups peanut butter

Instructions

In Instant Pot Select Sauté. Add coconut milk and honey. Cover your Instant Pot, set the vent to Sealing, select the manual or pressure cook button, select high pressure and set the timer to 3 minutes.

When done allow the pot to undergo natural pressure release for 15 mins.

Immediately stir in the marshmallow crème and peanut butter.

Pour and spread into a 9x9-inch glass baking dish. Cool completely before cutting into squares and serving.

Nutrition Facts

Calories 480, Total Fat 34.2g, Saturated Fat 8.4g, Cholesterol 0mg0%, Sodium 298mg, Total Carbohydrate 17.5g, Dietary Fiber 4g , Total Sugars 10.6g, Protein 16.3g

Matcha Avocado Pancakes

Preparation Time: 10 minutes Cooking Time: 5 min Servings: 6

Ingredients:

1cup Almond Flour

1 medium-sized Avocado, mashed1 cup Coconut Milk 1 tbsp Matcha Powder ½ tsp Baking Soda ¼ tsp Salt

Directions:

Mix all Ingredients into a batter. Add water, a tablespoon at a time, to thin out the mixture if needed. Lightly oil a nonstick pan. Scoop approximately 1/3 cup of the batter and cook over medium heat until bubbly on the surface(about 2-3 minutes). Flip the pancake over and cook for another minute.

Nutmeg Pears Small Balls

Prep time: 05 min Cooking Time: 30 min serve: 2

Ingredients

8 oz crescent rolls

1 small pears peeled, cored and cut into 8 wedges

1 tablespoon coconut oil

1/8 cup honey

¼ teaspoon vanilla extract

½ teaspoon ground nutmeg

Pinch ground cardamom

¼ cup red wine

Instructions

Open crescent rolls and separate into 2 triangles. Roll each wedge of pears in 1 crescent roll.

Add coconut oil to the Instant Pot. Use the display panel to select the Saute function.

When coconut oil is about Half melted, turn off the pot by selecting Cancel.

Add honey, vanilla and spices and stir until fully melted and incorporated. Add red wine and stir to combine.

Add dumplings in a single layer, then secure the lid, making sure the vent is closed.

Use the display panel, select the Manual or Pressure Cook function. Use the + /- keys and program the Instant Pot for 10 minutes.

When the time is up, let the pressure naturally release until the pin drops (for 15 minutes, whichever comes first).

Open the pot and let the dumplings cool and set for 3-5 minutes.

Remove dumplings and serve topped with any juices remaining in the pot.

Nutrition Facts

Calories 376, Total Fat 8.9g, Saturated Fat 6.4g, Cholesterol 1mg , Sodium 155mg, Total Carbohydrate

44g, Dietary Fiber 2.9g, Total Sugars 26.2g, Protein 3.5g

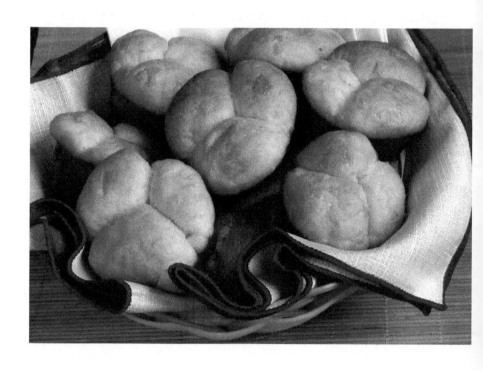

Lightning Source UK Ltd.
Milton Keynes UK
UKHW021306060521
383235UK00005B/114